Remembering Joey

Carla S. Moore

Remembering Joey

Copyright 2018 by Carla Moore
ISBN 9781790908585 Soft cover

All rights reserved
No part of this book may be reproduced or transmitted in any form or by any means, electronic or mechanical, including photocopying, recording, or by any information storage and retrieval system, without permission in writing from the copyright owner.

This book was printed in the United States of America.
To order additional copies of this book contact:
carla7191@att.net

FWB Publications
Columbus, Ohio 43207

FWB

Remembering Joey/ **Mentally Handicapped/Biography**

Remembering Joey

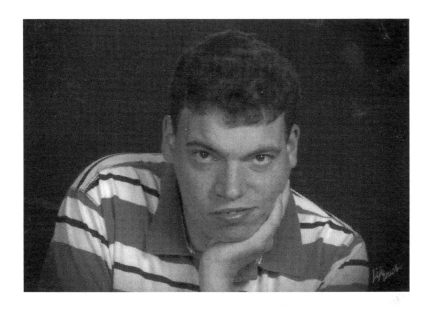

Joey

Dedication

I dedicate this book to my Mom. As Abraham Lincoln so eloquently stated "All I am or hope to ever be I owe to my Mom." I love you Mom and thank you for your love and support. I also dedicate the book to all Moms who are raising disabled children. May God help you, strengthen you and guide you as you care and love your precious gift.

Remembering Joey

Table of Contents

Preface 7

Introduction 9

Joey's Arrival 11

The Diagnosis 15

Childhood 19

Brain Surgery 25

Acceptance 29

Joey's Struggles 37

God's love extended to me and Joey 41

Joey's Death 45

God's Grace in my Darkest Hour 49

Epilogue 53

Remembering Joey

Remembering Joey

Preface

I wrote this book for the following reasons....

1) To educate people about individuals with disabilities, in hopes God reveals to them that they are truly the "perfect ones".

2) To honor the memory of my precious son, Joseph R. Wilder, whose impact will affect my life forever.

3) To share God's grace which has enabled me to put one foot in front of the other and continue on...

Remembering Joey

Remembering Joey

Introduction

Once in a lifetime God puts someone in your path that changes who you are forever. And as a result of their presence, you are a better person. For me that person was my special son Joey. Joey taught me some of the most valuable life lessons, and they are ones I will never forget. This story describes his journey and teaches the importance of acceptance of God's special children/adults. I hope this story will bless and inspire you to realize the gift of God's special people.

Carla S. Moore

(Joey's Mom)

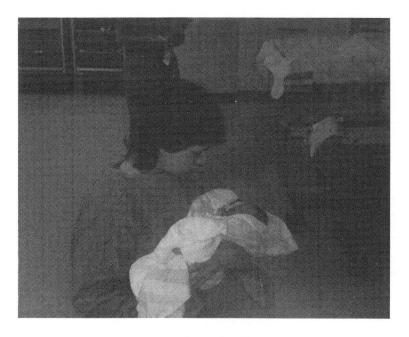

Joey's Arrival!

Joey's Arrival!

Psalm 127:3 Lo, children are an heritage from the Lord: and the fruit of the womb is his reward.

The day I found out I was pregnant with Joey was one of the most special days of my life! I was so excited! God was giving me this special gift! Me! I wanted to pinch myself to see if it was really happening. I believed motherhood was an important part of God's plan for me. I didn't realize just how important that plan would turn out to be.

I had been trying to get pregnant for 6 months and now after 9 months my baby was going to be born! I was so thrilled the day my son Joey was born! I'll never, ever forget that day. It was a hot August day in 1986. I was so excited about bringing this little bundle of joy into the world!

I'll never forget the first time I laid eyes on Joey. We bonded in a way I can only describe as a love that only God can orchestrate between a Mother and Child. He was mine and he was so beautiful and so perfect!

Remembering Joey

The first time I held Joey in my arms, he looked so deeply into my eyes...it was as if he wanted to say "Hey Mom! Your special little hero is here!" We named him Joseph Ryan Wilder. I recall thinking "That's a great doctor's name!" I had such high hopes for Joey. I also recall thinking, when I first held Joey "You're going to be someone special!" I didn't realize just how special Joey would turn out to be...

Joey struggled as an infant. At birth he weighed 8 lb 6 ½ oz and by one month he was up to 10 lbs! Then he developed a milk and soy allergy. After taking his formula he would projectile vomit. I kept telling his Pediatrician and he thought I was just a worried new Mom. He kept telling me that he was keeping down more milk than I thought. But I saw what was happening, I knew he couldn't be right. So I changed pediatricians only to find out by 3 months he was only 2 oz above his birth weight (8 lbs 8 oz)! Our new Pediatrician said Joey was nutritionally starved to death. I was so upset. No Mom wants to ever hear those words in relation to her new baby boy. How could this happen? I told the Pediatrician about my struggles to get his former Pediatrician to understand the extent of Joey's problem. I cried when I told him about it. Joey's Pediatrician told me later "Normally I would put infants who came to me in Joey's shape in the hospital but something told me that you would take great care of him." The Pediatrician put Joey on reglan and Nutramigen (which was a special formula without milk or soy-it was very expensive). I felt so sorry for Joey. The formula smelt like rotten potatoes.

Remembering Joey

I called the doctor and told him that Joey didn't like or want the formula. He told me to force it and eventually he would get hungry enough to take it. So I did. And Joey finally got to where he "liked" the formula and gained weight and appeared to be flourishing. Then he developed asthma...

When Joey's asthma would flair up he struggled to breathe. I would watch him and the entire bed would move up and down when he would breathe and it he made such a terrible rattling sound. We were in and out of Children's Hospital getting breathing treatments. The insurance company finally paid for a breathing machine. By about 6 to 8 months Joey outgrew the asthma. We were breathing a sigh of relief but little did we know what loomed on the horizon...

Remembering Joey

The Diagnosis
The Day My World Crumbled

Psalm 46:1 God is our refuge and strength, a very present help in trouble.

Joey was a wonderful loving baby. He brought such joy into our lives. I noticed whenever Joey awoke he would rhythmically jerk his head. It was just a slight movement but it always happened upon waking. I noticed it started the day after he received his first immunization. (I have since learned that 1 in every 100,000 infants will develop seizures as a result of the DPT vaccine. It's the Pertussis that causes the reaction. Joey never received the pertussis with his remaining immunizations, as his Pediatrician relayed it could make the seizures even worse). I mentioned what was happening to Joey upon awaking to his Pediatrician and he explained that often boys have immature nervous systems. I still had an uneasy feeling about it. (I believe God gives Mom's an instinct about their children. Don't ever doubt it. Trust it and find someone who will listen.)

The jerking became worse. And during a 6 month appointment while Joey was being examined for an ear infection and Joey had a "jerk" and his Pediatrician asked

Remembering Joey

"Is that what your son it doing?" I said "Yes". He said "Carla your son is having seizures. We need to get him to a Specialist." My beautiful baby boy...I was scared to death but was hopeful.

The day my world crumbed...I'll never forget that day. Joey was diagnosed with a seizure disorder, Lennox Gausteau Syndrome. I thought "Ok, we'll get him on medication and he will be fine." My optimism quickly diminished. Joey's Pediatric Neurologist relayed, "Joey has two types of seizures, infantile spasms and myocyclonic seizures. Both are the hardest to control. Left uncontrolled, Joey will become profoundly retarded." I fought back the tears and fell apart upon leaving the office. I felt as if my world was crumbling down all around me. My beautiful baby...all the hopes and dreams for his future are gone...no college, no marriage no grandchildren. What would happen to my precious child? I couldn't bear the thought...

To educate myself on Joey's condition I went to the main branch of the Columbus Public Library and checked out as many books as I could find on Joey's type of seizures. Everything I read indicated the children were severely mentally handicapped as a result of the disorder. I didn't understand God's plan. Where was God? I didn't want this for my son. How could I stop this fire that was taking my child's intellect? Please Lord help Joey! I felt my heart was breaking inside me.

Remembering Joey

I grieved for the longest time for the child Joey could have become. I spent many nights crying myself to sleep looking for answers...why? During this dark time in my life all I did was go through the motions...looking for answers...but there didn't appear to be any...

Remembering Joey

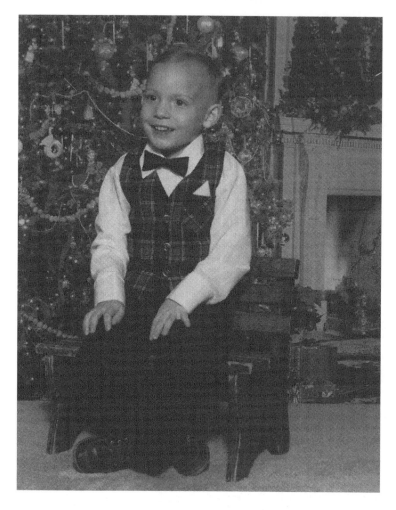

Childhood

Childhood

Matthew 18:4 Whosoever therefore shalt humble himself as this little child, the same is greatest in the kingdom of heaven.

Joey was put on medication in an attempt to control his seizures but nothing really helped. The seizures continued, but so did life. Joey was a <u>very</u> hyperactive toddler. He was very inquisitive and he was a bundle of energy! He always wanted to figure things out. Our Pediatrician told us if Joey would have been normal his IQ would have been a genius, but God had other plans.

We were blessed to have my precious Aunt Lottie and Uncle Norman babysit for Joey so that I could work. When Joey was there, their lives revolved around him. Aunt Lottie taught Joey his colors and his alphabet. He met the all normal growth milestones (walked at 12 months, learned to go to the restroom by himself by age 3, etc.). Uncle Norman would take Joey for walks in his little red wagon. They always wore their "fishing caps". Aunt Lottie said "I'd look out and there was Norman pulling Joey in a wagon and

Remembering Joey

both of them wearing their fishing hats." She said "It was comical!" Joey loved to play outdoors! (I guess he got that from me.) And on really hot days Uncle Norman had a fan in the garage he would turn on to keep Joey cool. Aunt Lottie always read to him. He had such a love for books. We would leave words out and Joey would fill them in. And if you "messed up" on a word he would tell you about it! And

I couldn't tell about his childhood without telling about his jeep. Joey loved his jeep! Santa brought it to him when he was 3 years old. It was a two-seater that ran on a battery. Joey continued to ride it until he was about 13 years old and could no longer fit in it! We had to change the tires 2 or 3 times because of his weight wore them down!

Joey loved going to the car wash. He would get SO excited! So Mom took the car to the car wash each week!

I believe if Joey had been normal he would have been a fireman or a policeman. He loved both of them. I had a friend who was a Fire Chief and he let Joey visit the fire station and sit in a fire truck. He was in the height of his glory!

He loved stuffed animals so much, we even buried him with his favorite one. Joey always had loads of "critters" in his bed. Before bedtime we had to make sure all of Joey's favorite "critters" were in his bed and we closed the night in prayer and Joey always prayed for kids with seizures like him.

Remembering Joey

Joey enjoyed the social aspect of school and won student of the month in a "regular" school he attended. When giving out the award the principal said "Joey has taught us much more than we have given him." Joey continued teaching us all of his life.

Joey also loved videos; Captain Kangaroo, PeeWee Herman and Barney the dinosaur were some of his favorites. He also loved to watch TV. I remember watching a show called "Rescue 911". It was about Paramedics. In this one episode a boy got his foot stuck in the toilet. One day I noticed Joey was taking a long time in the bathroom and I went in to check on him and low and behold he had his foot in the toilet! He was going to see if it would get stuck! Needless to say we monitored his television programs much closer after that!

And then were the funny things that come to mind like there was the time I bought a super large bottle (100 oz) of liquid Tide! And for some unknown reason Joey decided he was going to flush the entire thing down the toilet. When I went into the bathroom, the remaining drops were falling out of the bottle! Then there was the Vaseline encounter...one day we decided it was time to get Joey some walking shoes. So I put him in his car seat and on the floor was his diaper bag. Bad idea! When we pulled into the Stride Rite Store Joey was covered in Vaseline! It was in his hair and on his arms and legs! Needless to say we didn't buy any shoes that day! I had to scrub his head with Dawn dish detergent!

Remembering Joey

His poor head was red from the scrubbing!!! It makes me laugh just recalling it! He was so special and so full of life! And even though his seizures continued daily (60 to 100 a day) he always greeted each day with a smile. He was such a special blessing in our lives. I had no idea at the time where this seizure journey would take us...

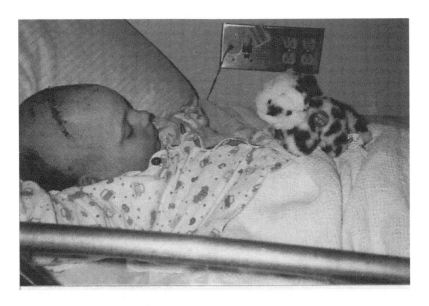

Brain Surgery

Remembering Joey

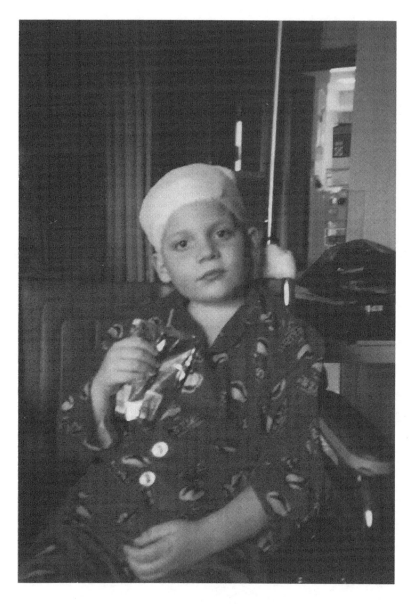

Brain Surgery

Brain Surgery

Psalm 22:11 Be not far from me; for trouble is near; for there is none to help.

The doctor's tried medication after medication to attempt to stop this burning inferno that was destroying my child. At the onset of this journey I felt in my heart that if I were Joey, I would want my parents to try everything thing that presented a glimmer of hope...and we did. I couldn't begin to tell you all the numerous medications that we tried. We'd try something new and get hopeful it would work, only to be disappointed. We even tried a ketogenic diet. Which involved simulating a fast, which doctors found improved some patients' seizures. Our lives revolved around Joey's medication schedule. And there were blood tests every 3 months to ensure the medication was not damaging his liver. (This routine would continue the rest of Joey's life.) Finally, the doctors recommended a brain surgery, corpus callosotomy. By this time Joey's seizures were coming from multiple places on both sides of his brain. They were so strong it would knock his legs right out from

Remembering Joey

under him. Once he fell and broke his ankle. By this time Joey was having 80 to 100 seizures a day. I wondered how much his little body could take. Life was so difficult for Joey. Why? With the corpus callosotomy surgery the surgeon would split Joey's brain stem and hopefully prevent the seizures from traveling through the brain stem and hopefully reduce their severity. We were told this would not be a cure for Joey's seizures, but they were hoping to reduce them by 50% and minimize their severity. We were also told everyone's brain is mapped different and they could cut into a major artery and it could result in Joey's death. It was a difficult decision but we felt God would take care of Joey.

The surgery was done in November of 1990. Joey was 4 years old. The surgery was 8 hours long. It seemed like an eternity. As a family we gathered in the Waiting Room and asked the Lord to guide the Surgeon's hands and help Joey. Joey came through the surgery with flying colors. For 3 days after the surgery Joey was seizure free. I couldn't believe the joy I felt and sense of a load being lifted from my shoulders. (If you have never had a handicapped child the stress is intense. There are constant worries and concerns. You can't let your guard down-they need you.) But my joy was short lived, the seizures returned the 4th day after surgery. The benefit we gained from the surgery was the fact that Joey now knew when the seizures were coming on and he would sit down to prevent injury. But the seizures continued….

Remembering Joey

When Joey turned 6 the doctors recommended another brain surgery to completely sever Joey's brain stem. (They only did it three-fourths of the way the first time. Again we prayed about it and asked God to watch over Joey and he did. But unfortunately the seizures continued. We had to wrap our minds around the fact that Joey's seizures were going to be a part of his life...whether we wanted the unwelcome guest or not...it was life, Joey's life. Joey's surgery and the results helped me start to accept the reality of his situation.

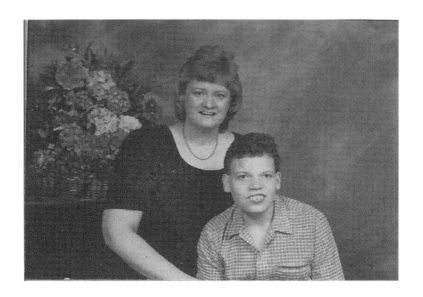

Acceptance

Acceptance

Proverbs 3:5 Trust in the Lord with all your heart and lean not on your own understanding;

No one ever "wants" their child to be profoundly retarded. As a parent you **only** want the best for them. I recall visiting with my parents asking, "Why doesn't God heal Joey?" I knew and believed He could do it, but why didn't he? Dad called a deacon friend over from his church at 10:00pm that night to talk with me. God used him to minister to me. He said to me "Susie perhaps this is the only way God can use Joey." Those words kept ringing over and over in my mind. I had to go to the door (figuratively) and open it and accept, love and treasure Joey for who he was...one of God's special children. I came to learn that God had a special plan for Joey's life and He used him in a mighty way. I think it is safe to say Joey left footprints on the hearts of all who knew him.

Joey offered everyone an unconditional love – it's similar to the love God offers each of us. Joey loved everyone. He never said anything bad about anyone.

Remembering Joey

Joey was a hard worker. Whether it was working on a sanding project for Grandma, vacuuming, cooking his mud and dirt stew or mowing the grass (which was a favorite activity).

Joey enjoyed eating. Especially mine and Aunt Lottie's mashed potatoes. His favorite restaurants were Bob Evans, the Olde Dutch Restaurant and Marcy's Diner. When he would arrive he'd say "Hey guys, I'm back!"

It wasn't always easy to care for Joey he had a strong will and was going to do what he wanted to do! (I guess he came by that honest too.)

Joey loved people and made them feel special in his special way. He loved to give out hugs and they came from deep within him. (Sometimes you thought he was going to love you to death (he didn't realize his own strength)!)

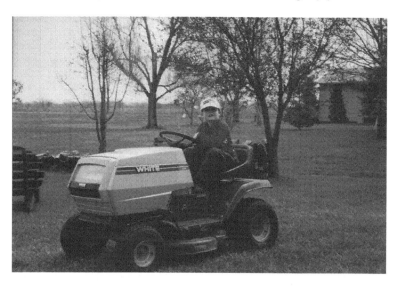

Remembering Joey

He was always picking my flowers to give to his Grandma, Aunt Lottie, or a favorite waitress or hairstylist. He always wanted to take my home canned apple butter and jams to his doctors and nurses. Needless to say he was the favorite patient!

Joey loved music (another trait he got from Mom)! Joey loved to hear me sing at church. He would get so excited! He'd say "Listen, it's Mom!" Christmas carols didn't have the same appeal as Joey loved them and listened to them from January to December. He also LOVED to hear Dolly Parton sing.

Joey loved to fish. Fishing provided him with an opportunity to spend time with Ernie (Joey's Step-Father), Grandma and Papaw. We went every Thursday. He instinctively knew it was "fishin' day" and he loved it!

Joey also loved camping. He always wanted to stay overnight and have a campfire. But when it got dark Joey's chicken feathers would come out and he would sit inside the camper with the light on and watch the campfire. In later years he wanted to go camping but at bedtime it was time for him and Mom to go home to our beds! ;)

Joey loved the computer and learned to operate it well. He had favorite games he would like to play.

Joey LOVED to vacuum! One day I couldn't locate Joey's shoes. I thought to myself "If I was Joey where would I hide my shoes."

Remembering Joey

I looked the house down, then the vacuum came to mind! Sure enough, he had zipped his shoes up in the sweeper bag! Try explaining to your boss you are late because your son hide his shoes in the vacuum bag and you liked to never found them!

He also LOVE mowing the lawn. A special friend let Joey mow her grass and he had went all over the yard, no pattern. Amy said "When a plane flies over they will think a UFO landed!"

Joey loved UPS trucks! He would get so excited when the "PS Man" delivered packages. He would have loved the fact that his Uncle Mark now works at UPS delivering packages!

Joey LOVED Christmas! From the carols, the tree, Santa, gifts (giving and receiving), lights, Christmas story of Baby Jesus. Everything about it!

He also LOVED family. He greeted everyone with a hug and unconditional love. That is what he was all about.

Joey dearly loved his dog Maggie. Maggie is a border collier and Australian Sheppard mix. She is such a gentle dog and loved Joey dearly. Joey loved to get a hold of her paws. I was constantly on to him to not hold them. Maggie didn't care for this either but she never retaliated; she would just look to me for help. Joey lived a full live and he loved it! Maggie reminds us so much of Joey. She has many of his personality traits.

Remembering Joey

Joey also loved church! I was blessed to have special friends who taught a Sunday School Class and they invited Joey to attend. He absolutely loved it and he enjoyed being with the other kids! We attended a Baptist church and my Father was a minister of the gospel. Often when the invitation to accept Christ was given and our Pastor would ask if anyone wanted him to pray that they would come to know Christ to raise their hand, Joey would often raise his hand. One Sunday evening Joey's Papaw was preaching and extended the invitation to come and accept Christ as your personal Savior, Joey went forward to the altar to pray. My Dad said he knew Joey understood what he was doing he could tell by the broken look on his face. We prayed with Joey as he accepted Christ into his life. Our Pastor said if Joey could see his need for Christ surely each of us could. What a blessing and comfort it is to me now. I look forward to the day when I get to heaven and meet Joey again. What a reunion! What a Savior!

If you were too died tonight would you go to Heaven? The Bible tells us in Romans 3:23 "That all have sinned and come short of the glory of God." We were born into sin through the sin curse of Adam and Eve's sin in the Garden of Eden. And Romans 3:23 tells us "For the wages of sin is death; but the gift of God is eternal life through Jesus Christ our Lord." Without Christ's redemption the wages for our sin is eternal punishment in Hell. But Roman's 5:8 tells us "But God commended His love toward us, in that, while we were yet sinners Christ died for us." Romans 10:13 "For whosoever shall call on the name of the Lord shall be saved."

Remembering Joey

Christ died for your sins. And Christ offers us forgiveness of those sins and eternal life in Heaven with Him. Do you want a personal relationship with Jesus Christ and the assurance of Heaven when you die? It is as simple as saying this prayer:

> Dear Heavenly Father,
>
> I am a sinner. I believe you died on the cross for my sins. I believe you were buried and arose on the 3rd day and are alive today and sit on the right hand of the Father. I repent of my sins and I ask you to come into my heart. Make we whole through the blood you shed on the cross for my sins. Help me live for you.
>
> In Jesus name.
>
> Amen

If you said this prayer, find a good bible believing church and attend faithfully.

It is my prayer that you grow in the grace and knowledge of our Lord Jesus Christ and one day you can meet Joey and I and our Lord in Heaven one day. I will forever be thankful for the blood of Christ that redeemed Joey and I and all who will come to Him.

Remembering Joey

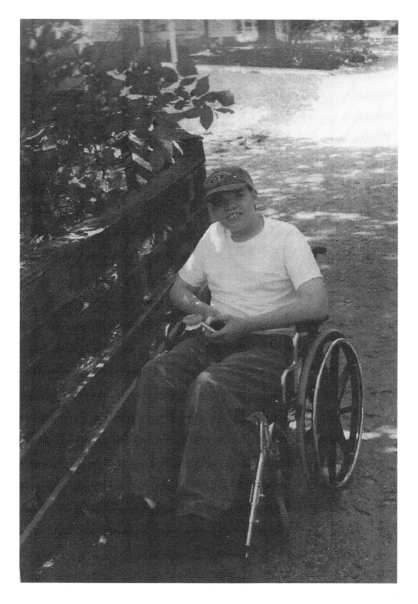

Joey's Struggles

Remembering Joey

Joey's Struggles

I John 4:4 You are of God, little children, and have overcome them; because greater is He that is in you, than he that is in the world.

Each person's life has difficulties and Joey's was no different. He struggled when my first husband and I divorced. It was hard for him to understand, but with time he accepted it.

One of the hardest things Joey experienced was Uncle Norman's death. They had such a special bond. Joey never wanted to talk about Norman after he died and it concerned me. One day him and Aunt Lottie were outside and he asked Aunt Lottie "Lod, where is Norm?" Aunt Lottie explained, "Norman died and he is up in Heaven beyond the clouds (she pointed up to the sky) and said he's watching you." That helped Joey accept Uncle Norman's death and he later opened up and talked about him. Joey, Lottie and I would decorate Norman's grave.

Remembering Joey

My Aunt Lottie developed Parkinson's Disease in the later years of her life and Joey saw her health deteriorate. When I would take Joey to visit Aunt Lottie she would light up. They had such a special connection. Joey never talked about it but I could tell by how he acted around Aunt Lottie it hurt him to see her sick. Lottie's death was also difficult for Joey to grasp. Joey passed away 3 weeks after Lottie. They wanted to be together.

The seizures took their toll and affected Joey's ability to walk. He had to wear braces. His Orthopedic Surgeon told me once that his legs have to be killing him, he has to be in constant pain...yet he never complained.

Joey knew Mom didn't like for him to say bad words. When Joey got angry he would say, "I'm going to say my bad word". And of course it came out at the most inappropriate places...like at church! I could have crawled under the pew!

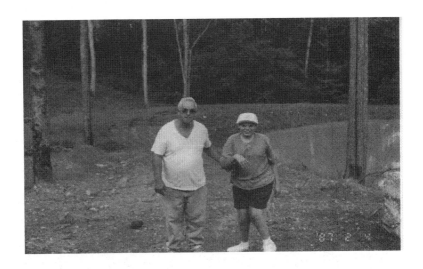

Remembering Joey

I recall Joey's Special Education Director telling me he loved that Joey was such a loving child. He said "Often they get mean and difficult as adults." The seizures took a toll on Joey's brain and deteriorated it. There were times when Joey would refuse to get out of our vehicle (of course it was usually on days where it was 90 degrees and 90% humidity). He'd be perspiring. He'd be so hot, but he wouldn't move! It seems funny now, but it sure wasn't at the time! He'd get frustrated easy and would bang his head on the walls or concrete side walk.

My husband had to repair the hallway and Joey's bedroom wall where Joey would get mad and put his fist through the wall. But my husband said "Joey has to get his frustration out somehow." But he never raised a finger to hit me. I don't say all these things to disgrace Joey's memory, in fact, I had no intension of telling these things but my husband said I should tell the good as well as the challenging times. I guess we all have these in our lives. One that seems so funny now was one summer day when it began to rain. Joey was in the backyard playing so I went out to bring Joey indoors.

He wasn't done playing. He flat out refused to come in. And when your child weighs 240 lbs it's hard to move him! By this time it is pouring down rain, thundering and lightening but Joey refused go in.

I had to call my Mom and she pretended to be a Police Officer and told Joey she was going to have to come get him if he didn't go inside with his Mom.

Remembering Joey

I'll be darned if Joey didn't get off the phone and walk right into the house! I had spent 30 minutes trying to coax him in! I don't regret any of the bad days. I loved Joey and when you love your children you accept the good with the bad.

God's Love Extended to Me and Joey

Philippians 4:19 And my God will supply all your needs according to His riches in glory by Christ Jesus.

I cannot fail to include God's love that was extended to us so graciously. So many blessing come to mind.

- **My Job** – I was blessed with an employer who provided me vast opportunities to pursue a fulfilling career. I was blessed with wonderful Managers who were so understanding to allow me to take off for Joey's doctor appointments and hospitalizations. Often my co workers were there with a listening ear during the bad times and some provided a shoulder to cry on. As a result, I gave 100% plus to my employer as a way to say thanks. The Bible instructs us to do our work as if unto the Lord. At times it was my job that provided a welcome refuge from the day's troubles and trials. It blessed me financially to provide the healthcare Joey needed and tremendous blessings!

Remembering Joey

- **My Family** – My loving Husband Ernie who was the Father he didn't have to be. Ernie was not only Joey's Step-Father, he was his best friend. He introduced so many things to Joey that he loved; fishing, sanding, building bird houses, camping. It was apparently the blessing God sent us when he gave us you. Each and every one of my family loved Joey and provided support for he and I. Joey dearly loved each of you and I'm sure he will be waiting at Heaven's gate to welcome and thank you for all you done for him and me. You all have a special place in my heart.
- **Special Friends** – Our special friends who loved Joey and made him feel special. In doing so, as the scripture says in Matthew 25:40. Inasmuch as ye have done it unto one of the least of these brethren, ye have done it unto me. I pray the Lord will bless you richly for it.
- **My Neighbors** – A neighbor mowed my grass for me and for weeks I never knew who did it. Another neighbor had her daughters remove the snow from my sidewalk and it would be clear when we arrived home. For the longest I had no idea who was doing it. Thanks to each of you for being Jesus to us.

Every need our Lord supplied. And he provided special blessings in those he used to be a blessing to us. All of these things are gifts and blessings from the Lord and I am thankful for them. What a blessing each of them were and are in my life.

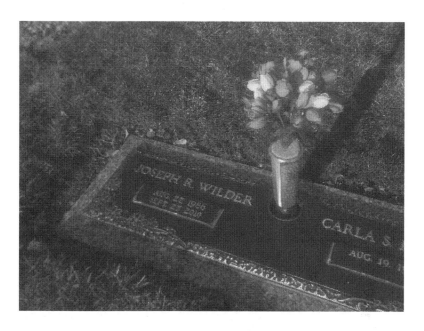

Joey's Death

Remembering Joey

Joey's Death

2 Corinthians 5:8 …to be absent from the body is to be present with the Lord.

I knew that one day I would have to face life without Joey. I would go to his bedroom door and think of this day but I had no earthly idea of the overwhelming loss I would experience. On September 26, 2010 Joey was hospitalized, the seizures were on their final attack. I stayed overnight with Joey and awoke around 2:00am and looked at Joey. He was laying there lifeless, he could not walk, talk or move. It was with tear-filled eyes I cried and prayed and told God this is not the life my Joey would want to live. It's ok with me if you want to take him. (Not that the Lord needed my approval but I believe he was preparing me for Joey's final hour.) The next morning September 27, 2010 at 10:00am Joey had the worst seizure I had ever seen. It involved his entire body. His entire body came up off the bed and his eyes rolled.

I recall saying "Oh my God, help him!" After the seizure was over Joey stopped breathing.

Remembering Joey

I grabbed his chest and rubbed it and said "Breathe Joey", and he'd breathe. I kept this up while screaming for a nurse. Joey was transported to Palliative Care in Intensive Care. I stood in a corner while the Doctors and Nurses worked on him and begged God to please heal him. Then I stopped and said "Lord I want your will to be in Joey's life."

You see I know God's will is perfect. The doctor came to me and asked me if I wanted to put Joey on life support. But he said there are no guarantees. We had just went through that with an Aunt of mine. She swelled up and everything.

I didn't want that for Joey but I didn't want to let my son go…I called my Mom and my ex-husband. Both told me only I could make that decision. I prayed and felt God telling me to release Joey. His healing would finally come. The Lord was merciful and I didn't have to make the decision.

I recalled the monitors going off and blood coming from Joey's mouth and ears. I screamed "I can't stand this!"

Then it donned on me what I say would be the last words Joey would hear from my lips. I put my fingers through his hair and told him over and over again "Joey I love you." My heart breaking with each word.

Then I just knew he was gone, I felt it. I had the nurse check. She said "I don't think so and she checked and she said "your right he's gone."

Remembering Joey

The bible teaches there is a time to be born and a time to die. On September 27, 2010 at 4:15pm Joey took his last breath and awoke in paradise.

God gave me such a peace about Joey's death. I knew in my heart he was now healed and in his creator's care. I even eulogized Joey at his funeral. I'm not sure how I did it. I can only tell you it was ONLY by God's grace.

At Joey's viewing there were 500 to 600 people. Joey had touched people's lives in a special way. You see I realized the day of Joey's funeral. Joey's life purpose was to share God's unconditional love with the world. Everything and everyone spoke of the special love Joey gave them. What better calling could anyone have on their life?

In Joey's death he taught me to live life to the fullest and to share God's love with everyone, they need it. Thank you Joey, for being my Joey, and for touching my life in such profound way. I was blessed to raise the best son ever. I look forward to our reunion one day.

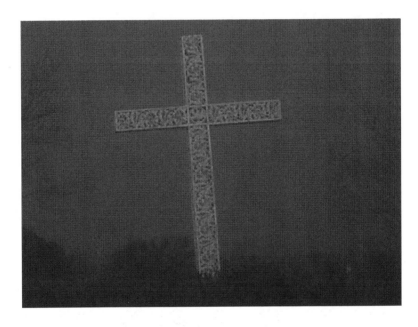

God's Grace in my Darkest Hour

God's Grace in my Darkest Hour

Matthew 28:20 ...and lo, I am with you always, even to the end of the world. Amen.

The bible teaches us that our days were written in his book. When God designed you he had a plan for your life and one day that life will be completed. Joey's work here on earth was completed on September 27, 2010. I have learned so much about myself and life through Joey's death. The Lord has taught me that I need Him each and every day, every hour of my life. In the good times and especially in the bad times. I trust Him with my life and pray He will accomplish His purpose in my life as he did in Joey's.

How do you go on when you lose your only son? By asking the Lord to help you put one foot in front of the other, that's how. He has proven His grace is sufficient and He promises to never leave me or forsake me and He has been faithful to that promise. Although Joey's life is over, mine isn't and to honor his life I will continue (with God's help) to finish my journey. I'll honor Joey's memory by doing the best with the gifts God has blessed me with.

Remembering Joey

I'll share unconditional love. I'll greet each day with a smile and one day I will meet my son in a place where seizures will never enter. Thank you Lord for blessing me with the special gift of Joseph Ryan Wilder. Joey thank you for loving me. Thank you Lord for your love, grace and mercy which will get me through anything I will ever experience in my life.

Remembering Joey....

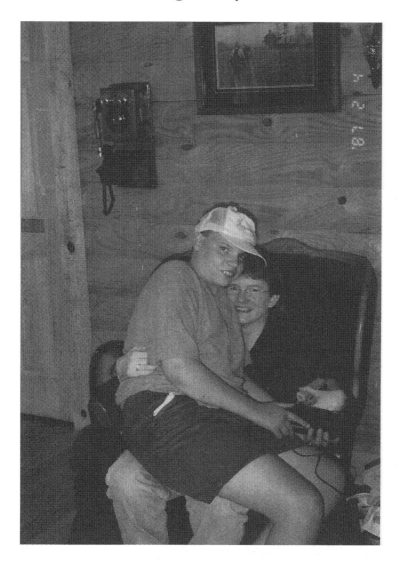

What a special gift...

Remembering Joey

Epilogue

This epilogue was written in 1996 when Joey was 10 years old. The Lord gave me this to help me accept Joey for who he was, one of His special children. I hope you enjoy "My Special Hero".

My Special Hero

The Birth of My Hero

I'll never forget the day my son Joey was born. It was a hot August day in 1986. I was so excited about bringing this bundle of joy into the world!

I'll never forget the first time I laid eyes on Joey. He was so beautiful and so perfect! The first time I held Joey in my arms, he looked so deeply into my eyes...it was if he wanted to say "Hey Mom! Your special little hero is here." We named him Joseph Ryan Wilder. I recall thinking "That's a great doctor's name! I had such high hopes for Joey. I also recall thinking, when I first held Joey in my arms, "Your going to be someone special!" I didn't realize just how special Joey would turn out to be...

The Day My World Crumbled

I'll never forget that day...Joey was diagnosed with a seizure disorder. I thought, "Ok, we'll get him on medication and he'll be fine." My optimism quickly diminished. Joey's Pediatric Neurologist relayed, "Joey has two types of seizures, infantile spasms and myoclonic seizures. Both are

Remembering Joey

the hardest to control. Left uncontrolled, Joey will become profoundly retarded." I fought back the tears and fell apart upon leaving the office. I felt as if my world was crumbling down all around me. My beautiful baby...all the hopes and dreams for his future were gone...no college, no marriage and no grandchildren.

I grieved for the longest time for the child Joey could have become. I spent many nights crying myself to sleep, wondering...why? During this dark period in my life all I did was go through the motions of everyday life...looking for answers...

Denial

The doctors tried medication after medication attempting to find some combination that would control Joey's seizures. But the epilepsy was like a fire burning out of control and slowly taking my child's intellectual capability. At one point, Joey was unable to verbally communicate, had no bladder control and we had to walk behind him to prevent him from falling and injuring himself. I still didn't want to accept Joey's situation. I wanted Joey to be normal...like other kids. I clung to the hope that we'd find the right combination of medication.

In 1991 Joey was referred to the Cleveland Clinic Foundation for a brain surgery evaluation...the reality was starting to settle in. On the way home from the Neurologist I looked over at Joey sitting beside me and was unable to hold back the tears...Joey reached over and gave me a hug and said, "Mom, why are you so sad?" I replied, "Honey, Mom's just worried about you." Joey replied, "Mom, I'll be ok." If only I could have Joey's faith, I could accept this.

Surgery

Joey had undergone two brain surgeries by the time he was 6 years old. The procedure involved severing Joey's brain stem. The theory was, split the brain stem and stop the seizures from traveling from both hemispheres of Joey's brain, thus reducing their severity.

By the time Joey underwent surgery, he was having over 100 seizures a day. Joey had no idea the seizures were coming on and the severity would knock the breath out of him. It made an awful sound. Joey would be sitting at the dinner table and the force of the seizures would cause Joey to land in his plate. Every time this would happen, I got a huge lump in my throat and could no longer eat. I was so scared that one day Joey would fall asleep, have a seizure, and never wake up.

The only way I made it through this time in my life was through the grace of God. I recall taking a large thermos of coffee into work so that I could make it through the day...Joey was waking up 8 to 10 times a night. But I held to the assurance that God never gives us more than we can handle.

Remembering Joey

Education

After Joey's surgery it was time to think about an education. Our school presented 2 options, place Joey in a multiple handicapped class in a public school setting or place him in the county's Mentally Retarded Developmentally Delayed Program (MRDD). Joey and I visited the MRDD program. The majority of the kids were confined to wheelchairs, in diapers and unable to verbally communicate. I just couldn't place Joey there. After visiting the program, I recall begging God to heal Joey. I didn't realize it at the time, but being at the MRDD program was forcing me to face reality.

Joey was placed in the multiple handicapped setting. Unfortunately, or maybe I should say fortunately, it didn't work out. During our final parent/teacher conference the Principal of the school suggested looking into placing Joey in a nursing home for the profoundly retarded. It was at that point God made me realize I had to start accepting Joey for who he is, not who he might become. I stood up to the Principal and announced, "I want to tell you something. God gave Joey to me, he's not "perfect" but he's mine and he's my responsibility. And as long as I have breath in my body I will see to it that Joey is taken care of.

Acceptance of my Special Hero

And the acceptance process began...loving and accepting Joey for who he is a very special child.

Remembering Joey

Joey's world is a world without hatred or prejudices. Joey has the unique opportunity to always be himself. He doesn't worry about what others think, or what they want him to be. Joey offers everyone an unconditional love. It's similar to the love God offers to each of us.

Joey has taught me to take time to enjoy the special things in life. One spring morning as we were headed out the door Joey exclaimed, "Mom the flowers are hatching!" One day I attended a breakfast at Joey's school. The teacher asked, "Joey would you like to show Mom how you do your job?" Joey got so excited. Joey's job was to collect the attendance sheets and take them down to the office. Joey would put an attendance sheet in his little basket and just smile and say "Mom, I'm doing my job!" It made me realize we all have a contribution to make and it's important to feel you are making a contribution to your world.

Joey's daily struggles have driven me to use my intellectual capabilities to the best of my ability. Joey offers everyone frequent hugs and "I love you's". His little smile lights up his entire face and brightens up the room. Think of how much better our lives would be if we could look at it through Joey's eyes. Of all people who have had an impact on my life, Joey's has been the greatest. Recently while watching Touched By an Angel Joey exclaimed, "Mom, I'm an angel too!" I told him "You sure are Joey, my angel on earth!

Today Joey is 10 years old and is attending our county's MRDD School. (Yes, it is the school I didn't want Joey to attend.) The school has been the best thing for Joey. It has made him so much more independent. The school's motto is "reaching beyond". They strive for the kids to reach beyond their disabilities and achieve all they can. Some kids win medals in Special Olympics, others learn to live independently and others even hold down jobs in the community. I'm the school's greatest cheerleader. I can't say enough about the wonderful things they do. I'm now chairing their Parent's Group.

My Hero and Others Like Him

By now you know my special hero is not a hero of a foreign war, a political figure or someone in the public eye. It's my special son Joey. Every night when Joey says his prayers, he prays for people like him.

The next time you see a mentally handicapped individual, offer them a smile. Keep them and their caregivers in your prayers and think of the special gifts people like Joey have to offer.

Written by: Carla Moore, Joey's Mother

Remembering Joey

Made in the USA
Columbia, SC
19 December 2018